SAY BYE BYE TO STRETCH MARKS

TAYO OYEBANJI

HOME REMEDIES FOR TREATING STRETCH MARKS

Copyright © 2012 Author Name

All rights reserved.

ISBN:

CONTENTS

1	Title Page	i
2	Copyright	ii
3	Dedication	iii
4	Introduction	iv
5	What is stretch marks	Pg 1
6	Causes of stretch marks	Pg 2-3
7	Importance of getting rid of stretch marks	Pg 4-5
8	Prevention of stretch marks	Pg 6-7
9	Home remedies for treating stretch marks	Pg 8-10
10	Medical treatments for stretch marks	Pg 11-13
11	Conclusion	Pg 14
12	About the author	Pg 15-18

DEDICATION

I dedicate this book to my daughters and wife and also to those who have been finding it difficult to live their normal life as a result of stretch marks. I want to assure you that the SOLUTION to your stretch mark problem has ended!

INTRODUCTION

Stretch marks are a common skin condition that affects both men and women, and they can occur on various parts of the body, including the abdomen, thighs, breasts, and arms. While stretch marks are not harmful to one's health, they can cause cosmetic concerns and may impact self-esteem. Fortunately, there are various ways to say goodbye to stretch marks, ranging from simple preventive measures to more advanced medical and surgical treatments. This eBook will explore several approaches to reducing the appearance of stretch marks, including prevention strategies, home remedies, medical treatments and surgical interventions. By understanding these different options, individuals can find the approach that works best for them and achieve smoother, more even-toned skin.

WHAT IS STRETCH MARKS

Stretch marks, also known as striae are streaks or lines that appear on the skin due to rapid stretching of the skin. They are a common skin condition that can affect men and women of all ages, although they are most commonly associated with pregnancy and rapid weight gain or loss. Stretch marks typically appear on the abdomen, hips, thighs, breasts, and arms and can vary in color from pink, red, or purple to white or silver. While stretch marks are not harmful to one's health, they can cause cosmetic concerns and may impact self-esteem.

CAUSES OF STRETCH MARKS

The primary cause of stretch marks is rapid stretching of the skin, which can occur due to various reasons. Some of the most common causes of stretch marks include:

Pregnancy: As the body undergoes rapid changes during pregnancy, the skin can stretch rapidly, leading to the development of stretch marks. Puberty: The body undergoes significant growth and hormonal changes during puberty, which can lead to stretch marks.

Weight gain or loss: Rapid weight gain or loss can cause the skin to stretch or shrink rapidly, leading to the development of stretch marks

Medical conditions: Certain medical conditions, such as Cushing's syndrome and Marfan syndrome, can cause the skin to stretch rapidly and lead to the development of stretch marks.

Genetics: Some individuals may be more prone to developing stretch marks due to genetic factors. While anyone can develop stretch marks, certain factors can increase the risk of developing them, such as being female, having a family history of stretch marks, and having a history of rapid weight gain or loss.

IMPORTANCE OF GETTING RID OF STRETCH MARKS

While stretch marks are not harmful to one's health, they can cause cosmetic concerns and impact self-esteem. Many individuals who develop stretch marks feel self-conscious or embarrassed about their appearance, particularly if they appear in visible areas such as the stomach or arms. This can lead to anxiety, depression, and a decreased quality of life. Getting rid of stretch marks can help to boost self-confidence and improve body image, leading to a more positive outlook and improved mental health. It can also allow individuals to wear clothing and engage in activities they may have avoided due to the appearance of their stretch marks. Furthermore, some individuals may find that their stretch marks cause physical discomfort or itching, particularly if they are raised or uneven. By treating or reducing the appearance of stretch marks, individuals can alleviate these symptoms and improve their overall comfort.

PREVENTION OF STRETCH MARKS

One can maintain a healthy diet through the following ways:
Eating a healthy, balanced diet can help to prevent stretch marks by providing the body with the nutrients it needs to maintain healthy skin. A diet rich in vitamin C, vitamin E, zinc, and silica can help to improve skin elasticity and reduce the risk of stretch marks. Foods such as fruits, vegetables, whole grains, lean protein, and healthy fats should be included in the diet to promote healthy skin.

Keep the body hydrated: Drinking plenty of water can help to keep the skin hydrated and prevent stretch marks. When the skin is hydrated, it is more elastic and less prone to stretching and tearing. It is recommended to drink at least 8-10 glasses of water per day to maintain optimal hydration.

Exercise: Regular exercise can help to maintain a healthy weight and reduce the risk of rapid weight gain or loss, which is a common cause of stretch marks. Exercise also helps to improve circulation, which can promote healthy skin and reduce the risk of stretch marks. It is recommended to engage in at least 30 minutes of moderate-intensity exercise most days of the week.

Avoid sudden weight gain or loss: Rapid weight gain loss can cause the skin to stretch or shrink rapidly, leading to the development of stretch marks. To prevent stretch marks, it is important to maintain a healthy weight through a balanced diet and regular exercise. Avoiding crash diets or rapid weight loss programs can also help to reduce the risk of stretch marks.

Gradual weight gain or loss is recommended, with a goal of losing or gaining no more than 1-2 pounds per week.

HOME REMEDIES FOR TREATING STRETCH MARKS

Aloe Vera gel: Aloe vera gel is a natural remedy that can help to reduce the appearance of stretch marks. It contains compounds that can help to promote skin healing and improve elasticity. To use aloe vera gel for stretch marks, apply a generous amount of fresh aloe vera gel to the affected area and massage it into the skin. Leave the gel on for at least 30 minutes before rinsing it off with warm water. Repeat this process daily for best results.

Coconut oil: Coconut oil is another natural remedy that can help to reduce the appearance of stretch marks. It contains fatty acids that can help to improve skin elasticity and reduce inflammation. To use coconut oil for stretch marks, apply a small amount of organic, unrefined coconut oil to the affected area and massage it into the skin in circular motions.

Leave the oil on overnight and rinse it off in the morning. Repeat this process daily for best results.

Vitamin E oil: Vitamin E oil is a powerful antioxidant that can help to improve skin health and reduce the appearance of stretch marks. To use vitamin E oil for stretch marks, break open a vitamin E capsule and apply the oil directly to the affected area. Massage the oil into the skin and leave it on for at least 30 minutes before rinsing it off with warm water. Repeat this process daily for best results.

Lemon juice: Lemon juice contains citric acid, which can help to exfoliate the skin and reduce the appearance of stretch marks. To use lemon juice for stretch marks, slice a fresh lemon and squeeze the juice onto the affected area. Gently massage the juice into the skin and leave it on for 10-15 minutes before rinsing it off with warm water.
Repeat this process daily for best results. Note that lemon juice may cause skin irritation in some individuals, so it is

important to test it on a small area of skin before using it on larger areas.

MEDICAL TREATMENTS FOR STRETCH MARKS

Retinoid creams: Retinoid creams are a type of topical medication that contains vitamin A derivatives. These creams can help to improve skin texture and reduce the appearance of stretch marks by increasing collagen production and improving skin elasticity.

Retinoid creams can only be obtained with a prescription from a dermatologist and should be used under their guidance.

Chemical peels: Chemical peels are a cosmetic procedure that involves applying a chemical solution to the skin to remove the outer layer of dead skin cells. This process can help to reduce the appearance of stretch marks by promoting collagen production and skin cell regeneration. Chemical peels can only be performed by a licensed professional and may require multiple sessions to achieve optimal results.

Microdermabrasion: Microdermabrasion is a non-invasive cosmetic procedure that uses a handheld device to exfoliate the outer layer of the skin. This process can help to reduce the appearance of stretch marks by promoting collagen production and improving skin texture. Microdermabrasion can be performed by a licensed professional and may require multiple sessions to achieve optimal results.

Laser therapy: Laser therapy is a medical procedure that uses high-energy pulses of light to target and remove damaged skin cells. This process can help to reduce the appearance of stretch marks by promoting collagen production and improving skin texture. Laser therapy can only be performed by a licensed professional and may require multiple sessions to achieve optimal results. It is important to note that laser therapy can be expensive and may not be covered by insurance

It is important to note that surgical treatments for stretch marks are invasive procedures that carry risks and require significant recovery time. These procedures may not be covered by insurance and can be expensive. Individuals considering surgical treatments for stretch marks should consult with a board-certified plastic surgeon to determine the most appropriate treatment plan based on their individual needs and goals.

CONCLUSION

Stretch marks are a common cosmetic concern that can be caused by a variety of factors, including pregnancy, weight fluctuations, and genetics. While it may not be possible to completely eliminate stretch marks, there are several ways to reduce their appearance and say "Bye Bye to Stretch Marks," ranging from prevention methods to advanced medical and surgical treatments.

Prevention methods include maintaining a healthy diet, staying hydrated, exercising regularly, and managing weight gain or loss. Home remedies such as aloe vera gel, coconut oil, vitamin E oil, and lemon juice can also be effective in reducing the appearance of stretch marks.

ABOUT THE AUTHOR

Tayo Oyebanji is an author, a producer, a digital strategist and also UNICEF Child Protection Result Based Manager who has dedicated his career to writing about body image and personal health. Tayo's latest project is a book about stretch marks, in which he seeks to educate and empower readers to improve the appearance of their skin and boost their confidence.

Tayo's interest in this topic stems from his research where people struggle with stretch marks, which developed during their teenage years due to rapid weight gain or some during pregnancy. He found that there was a lack of comprehensive information available on the subject and was determined help others in a similar situation.

Tayo has spent the past months researching and writing about stretch marks, drawing on the latest medical research and personal experiences of individuals who have successfully treated their stretch marks. His writing style is accessible and informative, using relatable anecdotes and easy-to-understand language to make complex topics more approachable. Tayo's book covers a range of topics related to stretch marks, including prevention, treatment, and future directions in research. He offers practical advice and resources for readers to improve their skin health. Tayo's work has been widely praised for its compassionate approach and empowering message. He is a sought-after speaker and has been featured in numerous media outlets. Overall, Tayo Oyebanji is a dedicated author and media strategist who has made it his mission to help individuals struggling with stretch marks feel more confident and comfortable in their skin as well as helping people in

HOME REMEDIES FOR TREATING STRETCH MARKS

their online business marketing challenges using different strategies to bring home sales for them. His book offers a comprehensive guide to this common issue, providing practical advice and support to anyone looking to improve their skin health.

TAYO OYEBANJI

www.ingramcontent.com/pod-product-compliance
Lightning Source LLC
Chambersburg PA
CBHW032312240526
45464CB00023BA/3000